IMPORTANT!

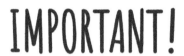

THIS BOOK IS TO HELP YOU COPE
BUT IT IS NOT MEANT TO REPLACE
PROFESSIONAL HELP

IF YOU ARE IN CRISIS, PLEASE SEEK
HELP OR CALL A CRISIS LINE FOR
IMMEDIATE ASSISTANCE.

INTERNATIONAL CRISIS LINES:

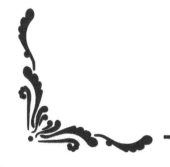

If you find this book helpful
please leave a review
on Amazon.
If you have any feedback you
can contact me at
howtobewiseaf@gmail.com

MORE BOOKS BY THIS AUTHOR

Gratitude & Wellbeing:

 The 90 Day Gratitude Habit Workbook Positivity | Mind and Soul practice Happiness, Mindfulness, Positivity, Affirmation, Self Care

The 90 Day Gratitude Habit Workbook For Grief: Three-month workbook for remembrance, gratitude & healing

Journaling:

 How To Be Wise AF Guided Journal For Women: A 30-day guided workbook for empowerment, strength, and resilience through good old-fashioned common sense and optimism

Problem Solving:

 What's Your Problem? Workbook For Women - Workbook -: A problem-solving journal with practical self-help exercises so you can figure it all out the next time the sh*t hits the fan

What's Your Problem? Workbook For Teens And Young Adults: A problem-solving journal with practical self-help exercises so you can feel more in control when life hands you a steaming pile of crap.

Car Maintenance:

 Car Maintenance & Repair Logbook For Women: All Your Car Care Information In One Handy Book: Maintenance Log & Checklists | Repair Research, History & ... Plan & Details Log | Reciept Saver Pouches

Fun Stuff:

The Serious Reader's Book Review Journal & Log Book | Journal For Book Lovers | 198 Page Reading Log -2 years of tracking, rating & reviews

 Describe It! For Writers | Creative Writing Prompts | Activity Book | Puzzles For Mental Stimulation | Fun Brainy Game: 101 Writing Prompts

 People I Have To Tell Off In The Morning And Excellent Come-Backs I Should Have Said Two Years Ago Notebook Lined Journal Diary Gift Joke Funny

Sketch, Dream Do | Sketch Book Composition Book | Great For Drawing, Sketching | For Artists, Doodling, Journaling

 Weird Dreams And Other Crazy Sh*t That Keeps Me Up At Night Bedside Journal Notebook Diary Lined Funny Gift: A bedside journal/book lined - sarcastic, funny cover

Caregiving:

 Eldercare Wellness Journal, Health Diary and Visit Log | Eldercare Health Record Book | Caring For Aging Parents | Reference Journal For Eldercare

Medical Notebooks:

 Personal Medical Notebook: Detailed Multi-Symptom Tracker | Personal Information Keeper | Doctor's Appointment Logbook

Medication Logbook & Personal Medical Notebook: Medication Logbook | Medical Information Keeper | Doctor's Appointment Logbook

 Blood Sugar Logbook & Personal Medical Notebook: 1 Year Blood Glucose Tracking Up To 6 Times Per Day | Medical Information Keeper | Doctor's Appointment Logbook

Blood Pressure Logbook & Personal Medical Notebook: Blood Pressure Logbook | Medical Information Keeper | Doctor's Appointment Logbook

 Chronic Pain & Symptom Diary/Journal - Health & Symptom Tracker Journal - Pain & Symptom Management - Medical Record Keeping - Healthcare - Wellness

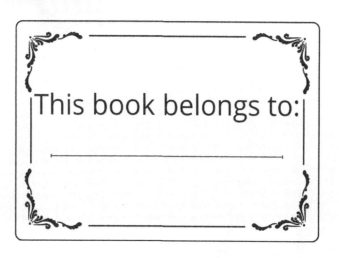

This book belongs to:

INSURANCE INFO

Company

Plan

Group #	ID #
Phone #	Contact

Company

Plan

Group #	ID #
Phone #	Contact

Company

Plan

Group #	ID #
Phone #	Contact

Company

Plan

Group #	ID #
Phone #	Contact

INSURANCE INFO

Company

Plan

Group #	ID #
Phone #	Contact

Company

Plan

Group #	ID #
Phone #	Contact

Company

Plan

Group #	ID #
Phone #	Contact

Company

Plan

Group #	ID #
Phone #	Contact

INSURANCE INFO

Company

Plan

Group #	ID #
Phone #	Contact

Company

Plan

Group #	ID #
Phone #	Contact

Company

Plan

Group #	ID #
Phone #	Contact

Company

Plan

Group #	ID #
Phone #	Contact

MEDICAL INFO
At a glance

NAME/ADDRESS   DATE/PLACE OF BIRTH   EMERG. CONTACTS

_____   _____   _____
_____   _____   _____
_____   _____   _____
_____   _____   _____
_____

HEIGHT/WEIGHT   ALLERGIES   EYE COLOR

_____   _____   _____

BLOOD TYPE   GLASSES PRESCRIPTION

_____   _____   _____

RECENT VACCINATIONS   MEDICAL CONDITIONS   DENTAL HISTORY

_____   _____   _____
_____   _____   _____
_____   _____   _____
_____   _____   _____
_____

MAJOR SURGERIES   MAJOR ILLNESSES   ALTERNATIVE THERAPIES

_____   _____   _____
_____   _____   _____
_____   _____   _____
_____   _____   _____

NOTES

MEDICAL INFO
Extra notes and information.

Family History

At a glance.

Mother's Side

_____
_____
_____
_____
_____

Father's Side

_____
_____
_____
_____
_____

Siblings

_____
_____
_____
_____

NOTES

EXTENDED MEDICAL HISTORY
Surgeries/Illnesses Etc

DATE	EVENT	DOCTOR	NOTES

EXTENDED MEDICAL HISTORY

Surgeries/Illnesses Etc

DATE	EVENT	DOCTOR	NOTES

EXTENDED VACCINATION LIST

Full vaccination history

DATE	VACCINE	DOCTOR	NOTES

MEDICATIONS LISTS
Lists of current medications & suppliments.

Name		Strength
Date started/finished	Form	Color/Shape
Reason for taking		How you take it
Prescribing doctor		Pharmacy

NOTES

Name		Strength
Date started/finished	Form	Color/Shape
Reason for taking		How you take it
Prescribing doctor		Pharmacy

NOTES

Name		Strength
Date started/finished	Form	Color/Shape
Reason for taking		How you take it
Prescribing doctor		Pharmacy

NOTES

		Strength
Date started/finished	Form	Color/Shape
Reason for taking		How you take it
Prescribing doctor		Pharmacy

NOTES

MEDICATIONS LISTS
Lists of current medications & suppliments.

NOTES

Name		Strength

Date started/finished	Form	Color/Shape

Reason for taking		How you take it

Prescribing doctor		Pharmacy

NOTES

Name		Strength

Date started/finished	Form	Color/Shape

Reason for taking		How you take it

Prescribing doctor		Pharmacy

NOTES

Name		Strength

Date started/finished	Form	Color/Shape

Reason for taking		How you take it

Prescribing doctor		Pharmacy

NOTES

		Strength

Date started/finished	Form	Color/Shape

Reason for taking		How you take it

Prescribing doctor		Pharmacy

MEDICATIONS LISTS
Lists of current medications & suppliments.

NOTES

Name		Strength
Date started/finished	Form	Color/Shape
Reason for taking		How you take it
Prescribing doctor		Pharmacy

NOTES

Name		Strength
Date started/finished	Form	Color/Shape
Reason for taking		How you take it
Prescribing doctor		Pharmacy

NOTES

Name		Strength
Date started/finished	Form	Color/Shape
Reason for taking		How you take it
Prescribing doctor		Pharmacy

NOTES

		Strength
Date started/finished	Form	Color/Shape
Reason for taking		How you take it
Prescribing doctor		Pharmacy

MEDICATIONS LISTS

Lists of current medications & suppliments.

NOTES

Name		Strength
Date started/finished	Form	Color/Shape
Reason for taking		How you take it
Prescribing doctor		Pharmacy

NOTES

Name		Strength
Date started/finished	Form	Color/Shape
Reason for taking		How you take it
Prescribing doctor		Pharmacy

NOTES

Name		Strength
Date started/finished	Form	Color/Shape
Reason for taking		How you take it
Prescribing doctor		Pharmacy

NOTES

		Strength
Date started/finished	Form	Color/Shape
Reason for taking		How you take it
Prescribing doctor		Pharmacy

MEDICATIONS LISTS
Lists of current medications & suppliments.

Name			Strength	**NOTES**
Date started/finished	Form		Color/Shape	
Reason for taking		How you take it		
Prescribing doctor		Pharmacy		

Name			Strength	**NOTES**
Date started/finished	Form		Color/Shape	
Reason for taking		How you take it		
Prescribing doctor		Pharmacy		

Name			Strength	**NOTES**
Date started/finished	Form		Color/Shape	
Reason for taking		How you take it		
Prescribing doctor		Pharmacy		

			Strength	**NOTES**
Date started/finished	Form		Color/Shape	
Reason for taking		How you take it		
Prescribing doctor		Pharmacy		

DOCTOR INFO

Family Doctor

Name

Address | Email

Phone # | Receptionist

Family Dentist

Name

Address | Email

Phone # | Receptionist

Specialist

Name

Address | Email

Phone # | Receptionist

Specialist

Name

Address | Email

Phone # | Receptionist

DOCTOR INFO

Specialist

Name

Address	Email
Phone #	Receptionist

Specialist

Name

Address	Email
Phone #	Receptionist

Specialist

Name

Address	Email
Phone #	Receptionist

Specialist

Name

Address	Email
Phone #	Receptionist

DOCTOR INFO

Specialist

Name

Address	Email
Phone #	Receptionist

Specialist

Name

Address	Email
Phone #	Receptionist

Specialist

Name

Address	Email
Phone #	Receptionist

Specialist

Name

Address	Email
Phone #	Receptionist

DOCTOR INFO

Specialist

Name

Address | Email

Phone # | Receptionist

Specialist

Name

Address | Email

Phone # | Receptionist

Specialist

Name

Address | Email

Phone # | Receptionist

Specialist

Name

Address | Email

Phone # | Receptionist

DOCTOR INFO

Specialist

Name

Address	Email
Phone #	Receptionist

Specialist

Name

Address	Email
Phone #	Receptionist

Specialist

Name

Address	Email
Phone #	Receptionist

Specialist

Name

Address	Email
Phone #	Receptionist

Symptom Tracker At A Glance

Check off the days that you have symptoms.

Month/Year _____

Notes: _____

_____

_____

_____

Mo	Tu	We	Th	Fr	Sa	Su

Month/Year _____

Notes: _____

_____

_____

_____

Mo	Tu	We	Th	Fr	Sa	Su

Month/Year _____

Notes: _____

_____

_____

_____

Mo	Tu	We	Th	Fr	Sa	Su

Month/Year _____

Notes: _____

_____

_____

_____

Mo	Tu	We	Th	Fr	Sa	Su

Symptom Tracker At A Glance

Check off the days that you have symptoms.

	Mo	Tu	We	Th	Fr	Sa	Su

Month/Year _____

Notes: _____

_____

_____

_____

_____

	Mo	Tu	We	Th	Fr	Sa	Su

Month/Year _____

Notes: _____

_____

_____

_____

_____

	Mo	Tu	We	Th	Fr	Sa	Su

Month/Year _____

Notes: _____

_____

_____

_____

_____

	Mo	Tu	We	Th	Fr	Sa	Su

Month/Year _____

Notes: _____

_____

_____

_____

_____

Symptom Tracker At A Glance

Check off the days that you have symptoms.

Month/Year _____

Notes: _____

_____

_____

_____

Mo	Tu	We	Th	Fr	Sa	Su

Month/Year _____

Notes: _____

_____

_____

_____

Mo	Tu	We	Th	Fr	Sa	Su

Month/Year _____

Notes: _____

_____

_____

_____

Mo	Tu	We	Th	Fr	Sa	Su

Month/Year _____

Notes: _____

_____

_____

_____

Mo	Tu	We	Th	Fr	Sa	Su

Symptom Tracker At A Glance
Check off the days that you have symptoms.

	Mo	Tu	We	Th	Fr	Sa	Su

Month/Year _____

Notes: _____

_____

_____

_____

	Mo	Tu	We	Th	Fr	Sa	Su

Month/Year _____

Notes: _____

_____

_____

_____

	Mo	Tu	We	Th	Fr	Sa	Su

Month/Year _____

Notes: _____

_____

_____

_____

	Mo	Tu	We	Th	Fr	Sa	Su

Month/Year _____

Notes: _____

_____

_____

_____

Symptom Tracker At A Glance

Check off the days that you have symptoms.

Month/Year _____

	Mo	Tu	We	Th	Fr	Sa	Su

Notes: _____

_____

_____

_____

Month/Year _____

	Mo	Tu	We	Th	Fr	Sa	Su

Notes: _____

_____

_____

_____

Month/Year _____

	Mo	Tu	We	Th	Fr	Sa	Su

Notes: _____

_____

_____

_____

Month/Year _____

	Mo	Tu	We	Th	Fr	Sa	Su

Notes: _____

_____

_____

_____

Symptom Tracker At A Glance

Check off the days that you have symptoms.

Month/Year _____

Notes: _____

_____

_____

_____

Mo	Tu	We	Th	Fr	Sa	Su
○	○	○	○	○	○	○
○	○	○	○	○	○	○
○	○	○	○	○	○	○
○	○	○	○	○	○	○
○	○	○	○	○	○	○

Month/Year _____

Notes: _____

_____

_____

_____

Mo	Tu	We	Th	Fr	Sa	Su
○	○	○	○	○	○	○
○	○	○	○	○	○	○
○	○	○	○	○	○	○
○	○	○	○	○	○	○
○	○	○	○	○	○	○

Month/Year _____

Notes: _____

_____

_____

_____

Mo	Tu	We	Th	Fr	Sa	Su
○	○	○	○	○	○	○
○	○	○	○	○	○	○
○	○	○	○	○	○	○
○	○	○	○	○	○	○
○	○	○	○	○	○	○

Month/Year _____

Notes: _____

_____

_____

_____

Mo	Tu	We	Th	Fr	Sa	Su
○	○	○	○	○	○	○
○	○	○	○	○	○	○
○	○	○	○	○	○	○
○	○	○	○	○	○	○
○	○	○	○	○	○	○

Symptom Tracker

_____

ENERGY LEVEL **TODAY'S MOOD** **WEATHER**

(1) (2) (3) (4) (5)

time	symptom	trigger	severity	duration
			1 2 3 4 5	
			1 2 3 4 5	
			1 2 3 4 5	
			1 2 3 4 5	
			1 2 3 4 5	
			1 2 3 4 5	
			1 2 3 4 5	
			1 2 3 4 5	
			1 2 3 4 5	
			1 2 3 4 5	

Notes

Breakfast

Lunch

Dinner

Water

SHOW ME WHERE IT HURTS: FRONT   **SHOW ME WHERE IT HURTS: BACK**

MEDICATION & SUPPLIMENTS

DOSAGE	NAME	TIME

Symptom Tracker

_____

ENERGY LEVEL

(1) (2) (3) (4) (5)

TODAY'S MOOD

WEATHER

time	symptom	trigger	severity	duration
			1 2 3 4 5	
			1 2 3 4 5	
			1 2 3 4 5	
			1 2 3 4 5	
			1 2 3 4 5	
			1 2 3 4 5	
			1 2 3 4 5	
			1 2 3 4 5	
			1 2 3 4 5	
			1 2 3 4 5	

Notes

Breakfast

Lunch

Dinner

Water +

SHOW ME WHERE IT HURTS: FRONT

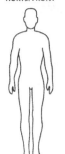

SHOW ME WHERE IT HURTS: BACK

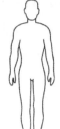

MEDICATION & SUPPLIMENTS

DOSAGE	NAME	TIME

Symptom Tracker

ENERGY LEVEL

(1) (2) (3) (4) (5)

TODAY'S MOOD

WEATHER

time	symptom	trigger	severity	duration
			1 2 3 4 5	
			1 2 3 4 5	
			1 2 3 4 5	
			1 2 3 4 5	
			1 2 3 4 5	
			1 2 3 4 5	
			1 2 3 4 5	
			1 2 3 4 5	
			1 2 3 4 5	
			1 2 3 4 5	

Notes

Breakfast

Lunch

Dinner

Water 🥛🥛🥛🥛🥛🥛🥛 +

SHOW ME WHERE IT HURTS: FRONT

SHOW ME WHERE IT HURTS: BACK

MEDICATION & SUPPLIMENTS

DOSAGE	NAME	TIME

Symptom Tracker

ENERGY LEVEL

(1) (2) (3) (4) (5)

TODAY'S MOOD

WEATHER

time	symptom	trigger	severity	duration
			1 2 3 4 5	
			1 2 3 4 5	
			1 2 3 4 5	
			1 2 3 4 5	
			1 2 3 4 5	
			1 2 3 4 5	
			1 2 3 4 5	
			1 2 3 4 5	
			1 2 3 4 5	
			1 2 3 4 5	

Notes

Breakfast

Lunch

Dinner

Water   +

SHOW ME WHERE IT HURTS: FRONT

SHOW ME WHERE IT HURTS: BACK

MEDICATION & SUPPLIMENTS

DOSAGE	NAME	TIME

Symptom Tracker

ENERGY LEVEL

(1) (2) (3) (4) (5)

TODAY'S MOOD

WEATHER

time	symptom	trigger	severity	duration
			1 2 3 4 5	
			1 2 3 4 5	
			1 2 3 4 5	
			1 2 3 4 5	
			1 2 3 4 5	
			1 2 3 4 5	
			1 2 3 4 5	
			1 2 3 4 5	
			1 2 3 4 5	
			1 2 3 4 5	

Notes

Breakfast

Lunch

Dinner

Water ▢ ▢ ▢ ▢ ▢ ▢ ▢ +

SHOW ME WHERE IT HURTS: FRONT

SHOW ME WHERE IT HURTS: BACK

MEDICATION & SUPPLIMENTS

DOSAGE	NAME	TIME

Symptom Tracker

ENERGY LEVEL

(1)(2)(3)(4)(5)

TODAY'S MOOD

WEATHER

time	symptom	trigger	severity	duration
			1 2 3 4 5	
			1 2 3 4 5	
			1 2 3 4 5	
			1 2 3 4 5	
			1 2 3 4 5	
			1 2 3 4 5	
			1 2 3 4 5	
			1 2 3 4 5	
			1 2 3 4 5	
			1 2 3 4 5	

Notes

Breakfast

Lunch

Dinner

Water +

SHOW ME WHERE IT HURTS: FRONT

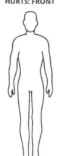

SHOW ME WHERE IT HURTS: BACK

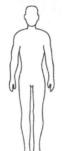

MEDICATION & SUPPLIMENTS

DOSAGE	NAME	TIME

Symptom Tracker

ENERGY LEVEL

(1) (2) (3) (4) (5)

TODAY'S MOOD

WEATHER

time	symptom	trigger	severity	duration
			1 2 3 4 5	
			1 2 3 4 5	
			1 2 3 4 5	
			1 2 3 4 5	
			1 2 3 4 5	
			1 2 3 4 5	
			1 2 3 4 5	
			1 2 3 4 5	
			1 2 3 4 5	
			1 2 3 4 5	

Notes

Breakfast

Lunch

Dinner

Water

SHOW ME WHERE IT HURTS: FRONT

SHOW ME WHERE IT HURTS: BACK

MEDICATION & SUPPLIMENTS

DOSAGE	NAME	TIME

Symptom Tracker

ENERGY LEVEL

(1) (2) (3) (4) (5)

TODAY'S MOOD

WEATHER

time	symptom	trigger	severity	duration
			1 2 3 4 5	
			1 2 3 4 5	
			1 2 3 4 5	
			1 2 3 4 5	
			1 2 3 4 5	
			1 2 3 4 5	
			1 2 3 4 5	
			1 2 3 4 5	
			1 2 3 4 5	
			1 2 3 4 5	

Notes

Breakfast

Lunch

Dinner

Water

SHOW ME WHERE IT HURTS: FRONT

SHOW ME WHERE IT HURTS: BACK

MEDICATION & SUPPLIMENTS

DOSAGE	NAME	TIME

Symptom Tracker

_____

ENERGY LEVEL

(1) (2) (3) (4) (5)

TODAY'S MOOD

WEATHER

time	symptom	trigger	severity	duration
			1 2 3 4 5	
			1 2 3 4 5	
			1 2 3 4 5	
			1 2 3 4 5	
			1 2 3 4 5	
			1 2 3 4 5	
			1 2 3 4 5	
			1 2 3 4 5	
			1 2 3 4 5	
			1 2 3 4 5	

Notes

Breakfast

Lunch

Dinner

Water

SHOW ME WHERE IT HURTS: FRONT

SHOW ME WHERE IT HURTS: BACK

MEDICATION & SUPPLIMENTS

DOSAGE	NAME	TIME

Symptom Tracker

ENERGY LEVEL   **TODAY'S MOOD**   **WEATHER**

(1) (2) (3) (4) (5)

time	symptom	trigger	severity	duration
			1 2 3 4 5	
			1 2 3 4 5	
			1 2 3 4 5	
			1 2 3 4 5	
			1 2 3 4 5	
			1 2 3 4 5	
			1 2 3 4 5	
			1 2 3 4 5	
			1 2 3 4 5	
			1 2 3 4 5	

Notes

Breakfast

Lunch

Dinner

Water

SHOW ME WHERE IT HURTS: FRONT   **SHOW ME WHERE IT HURTS: BACK**

MEDICATION & SUPPLIMENTS

DOSAGE	NAME	TIME

Symptom Tracker

DATE
_____

ENERGY LEVEL

(1) (2) (3) (4) (5)

TODAY'S MOOD

WEATHER

time	symptom	trigger	severity	duration
			1 2 3 4 5	
			1 2 3 4 5	
			1 2 3 4 5	
			1 2 3 4 5	
			1 2 3 4 5	
			1 2 3 4 5	
			1 2 3 4 5	
			1 2 3 4 5	
			1 2 3 4 5	
			1 2 3 4 5	

Notes

Breakfast

Lunch

Dinner

Water 🥛 🥛 🥛 🥛 🥛 🥛 🥛 +

SHOW ME WHERE IT HURTS: FRONT

SHOW ME WHERE IT HURTS: BACK

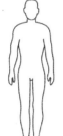

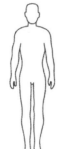

MEDICATION & SUPPLIMENTS

DOSAGE	NAME	TIME

Symptom Tracker

ENERGY LEVEL

(1) (2) (3) (4) (5)

TODAY'S MOOD

WEATHER

time	symptom	trigger	severity	duration
			1 2 3 4 5	
			1 2 3 4 5	
			1 2 3 4 5	
			1 2 3 4 5	
			1 2 3 4 5	
			1 2 3 4 5	
			1 2 3 4 5	
			1 2 3 4 5	
			1 2 3 4 5	
			1 2 3 4 5	

Notes

Breakfast

Lunch

Dinner

Water ⬜ ⬜ ⬜ ⬜ ⬜ ⬜ ⬜ +

SHOW ME WHERE IT HURTS: FRONT

SHOW ME WHERE IT HURTS: BACK

MEDICATION & SUPPLIMENTS

DOSAGE	NAME	TIME

Symptom Tracker

ENERGY LEVEL

(1) (2) (3) (4) (5)

TODAY'S MOOD

WEATHER

time	symptom	trigger	severity	duration
			1 2 3 4 5	
			1 2 3 4 5	
			1 2 3 4 5	
			1 2 3 4 5	
			1 2 3 4 5	
			1 2 3 4 5	
			1 2 3 4 5	
			1 2 3 4 5	
			1 2 3 4 5	
			1 2 3 4 5	

Notes

Breakfast

Lunch

Dinner

Water

SHOW ME WHERE IT HURTS: FRONT

SHOW ME WHERE IT HURTS: BACK

MEDICATION & SUPPLIMENTS

DOSAGE	NAME	TIME

Symptom Tracker

ENERGY LEVEL

(1) (2) (3) (4) (5)

TODAY'S MOOD

WEATHER

time	symptom	trigger	severity	duration
			1 2 3 4 5	
			1 2 3 4 5	
			1 2 3 4 5	
			1 2 3 4 5	
			1 2 3 4 5	
			1 2 3 4 5	
			1 2 3 4 5	
			1 2 3 4 5	
			1 2 3 4 5	
			1 2 3 4 5	

Notes

Breakfast

Lunch

Dinner

Water

SHOW ME WHERE IT
HURTS: FRONT

SHOW ME WHERE IT
HURTS: BACK

MEDICATION & SUPPLIMENTS

DOSAGE	NAME	TIME

Symptom Tracker

ENERGY LEVEL

(1) (2) (3) (4) (5)

TODAY'S MOOD

WEATHER

time	symptom	trigger	severity	duration
			1 2 3 4 5	
			1 2 3 4 5	
			1 2 3 4 5	
			1 2 3 4 5	
			1 2 3 4 5	
			1 2 3 4 5	
			1 2 3 4 5	
			1 2 3 4 5	
			1 2 3 4 5	
			1 2 3 4 5	

Notes

Breakfast

Lunch

Dinner

Water

SHOW ME WHERE IT
HURTS: FRONT

SHOW ME WHERE IT
HURTS: BACK

MEDICATION & SUPPLIMENTS

DOSAGE	NAME	TIME

Symptom Tracker

ENERGY LEVEL   TODAY'S MOOD   WEATHER

(1) (2) (3) (4) (5)

time	symptom	trigger	severity	duration
			1 2 3 4 5	
			1 2 3 4 5	
			1 2 3 4 5	
			1 2 3 4 5	
			1 2 3 4 5	
			1 2 3 4 5	
			1 2 3 4 5	
			1 2 3 4 5	
			1 2 3 4 5	
			1 2 3 4 5	

Notes

Breakfast

Lunch

Dinner

Water   🥛 🥛 🥛 🥛 🥛 🥛 🥛 +

SHOW ME WHERE IT
HURTS: FRONT

SHOW ME WHERE IT
HURTS: BACK

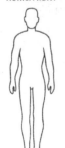
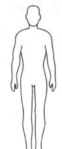

MEDICATION
& SUPPLIMENTS

DOSAGE	NAME	TIME

Symptom Tracker

ENERGY LEVEL

(1) (2) (3) (4) (5)

TODAY'S MOOD

WEATHER

time	symptom	trigger	severity	duration
			1 2 3 4 5	
			1 2 3 4 5	
			1 2 3 4 5	
			1 2 3 4 5	
			1 2 3 4 5	
			1 2 3 4 5	
			1 2 3 4 5	
			1 2 3 4 5	
			1 2 3 4 5	
			1 2 3 4 5	

Notes

Breakfast

Lunch

Dinner

Water

SHOW ME WHERE IT HURTS: FRONT

SHOW ME WHERE IT HURTS: BACK

MEDICATION & SUPPLIMENTS

DOSAGE	NAME	TIME

Symptom Tracker

ENERGY LEVEL

(1) (2) (3) (4) (5)

TODAY'S MOOD

WEATHER

time	symptom	trigger	severity	duration
			1 2 3 4 5	
			1 2 3 4 5	
			1 2 3 4 5	
			1 2 3 4 5	
			1 2 3 4 5	
			1 2 3 4 5	
			1 2 3 4 5	
			1 2 3 4 5	
			1 2 3 4 5	
			1 2 3 4 5	

Notes

Breakfast

Lunch

Dinner

Water 🥛🥛🥛🥛🥛🥛🥛 +

SHOW ME WHERE IT HURTS: FRONT

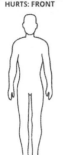

SHOW ME WHERE IT HURTS: BACK

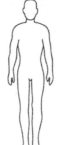

MEDICATION & SUPPLIMENTS

DOSAGE	NAME	TIME

Symptom Tracker

ENERGY LEVEL   **TODAY'S MOOD**   **WEATHER**

(1) (2) (3) (4) (5)

time	symptom	trigger	severity	duration
			1 2 3 4 5	
			1 2 3 4 5	
			1 2 3 4 5	
			1 2 3 4 5	
			1 2 3 4 5	
			1 2 3 4 5	
			1 2 3 4 5	
			1 2 3 4 5	
			1 2 3 4 5	
			1 2 3 4 5	

Notes

Breakfast

Lunch

Dinner

Water   +

SHOW ME WHERE IT HURTS: FRONT   **SHOW ME WHERE IT HURTS: BACK**

MEDICATION & SUPPLIMENTS

DOSAGE	NAME	TIME

Symptom Tracker

ENERGY LEVEL

(1) (2) (3) (4) (5)

TODAY'S MOOD

WEATHER

time	symptom	trigger	severity	duration
			1 2 3 4 5	
			1 2 3 4 5	
			1 2 3 4 5	
			1 2 3 4 5	
			1 2 3 4 5	
			1 2 3 4 5	
			1 2 3 4 5	
			1 2 3 4 5	
			1 2 3 4 5	
			1 2 3 4 5	

Notes

Breakfast

Lunch

Dinner

Water +

SHOW ME WHERE IT HURTS: FRONT

SHOW ME WHERE IT HURTS: BACK

MEDICATION & SUPPLIMENTS

DOSAGE	NAME	TIME

Symptom Tracker

_____

ENERGY LEVEL

(1) (2) (3) (4) (5)

TODAY'S MOOD

WEATHER

time	symptom	trigger	severity	duration
			1 2 3 4 5	
			1 2 3 4 5	
			1 2 3 4 5	
			1 2 3 4 5	
			1 2 3 4 5	
			1 2 3 4 5	
			1 2 3 4 5	
			1 2 3 4 5	
			1 2 3 4 5	
			1 2 3 4 5	

Notes

Breakfast

Lunch

Dinner

Water ☐ ☐ ☐ ☐ ☐ ☐ ☐ +

SHOW ME WHERE IT HURTS: FRONT

SHOW ME WHERE IT HURTS: BACK

MEDICATION & SUPPLIMENTS

DOSAGE	NAME	TIME

Symptom Tracker

ENERGY LEVEL

(1) (2) (3) (4) (5)

TODAY'S MOOD

WEATHER

time	symptom	trigger	severity	duration
			1 2 3 4 5	
			1 2 3 4 5	
			1 2 3 4 5	
			1 2 3 4 5	
			1 2 3 4 5	
			1 2 3 4 5	
			1 2 3 4 5	
			1 2 3 4 5	
			1 2 3 4 5	
			1 2 3 4 5	

Notes

Breakfast

Lunch

Dinner

Water +

SHOW ME WHERE IT HURTS: FRONT

SHOW ME WHERE IT HURTS: BACK

MEDICATION & SUPPLIMENTS

DOSAGE	NAME	TIME

Symptom Tracker

ENERGY LEVEL

(1) (2) (3) (4) (5)

TODAY'S MOOD

WEATHER

time	symptom	trigger	severity	duration
			1 2 3 4 5	
			1 2 3 4 5	
			1 2 3 4 5	
			1 2 3 4 5	
			1 2 3 4 5	
			1 2 3 4 5	
			1 2 3 4 5	
			1 2 3 4 5	
			1 2 3 4 5	
			1 2 3 4 5	

Notes

Breakfast

Lunch

Dinner

Water ▢ ▢ ▢ ▢ ▢ ▢ ▢ +

SHOW ME WHERE IT HURTS: FRONT

SHOW ME WHERE IT HURTS: BACK

MEDICATION & SUPPLIMENTS

DOSAGE	NAME	TIME

Symptom Tracker

ENERGY LEVEL

(1) (2) (3) (4) (5)

TODAY'S MOOD

WEATHER

time	symptom	trigger	severity	duration
			1 2 3 4 5	
			1 2 3 4 5	
			1 2 3 4 5	
			1 2 3 4 5	
			1 2 3 4 5	
			1 2 3 4 5	
			1 2 3 4 5	
			1 2 3 4 5	
			1 2 3 4 5	
			1 2 3 4 5	

Notes

Breakfast

Lunch

Dinner

Water ⊔ ⊔ ⊔ ⊔ ⊔ ⊔ +

SHOW ME WHERE IT HURTS: FRONT

SHOW ME WHERE IT HURTS: BACK

MEDICATION & SUPPLIMENTS

DOSAGE	NAME	TIME

Symptom Tracker

_____

ENERGY LEVEL

(1) (2) (3) (4) (5)

TODAY'S MOOD

WEATHER

time	symptom	trigger	severity	duration
			1 2 3 4 5	
			1 2 3 4 5	
			1 2 3 4 5	
			1 2 3 4 5	
			1 2 3 4 5	
			1 2 3 4 5	
			1 2 3 4 5	
			1 2 3 4 5	
			1 2 3 4 5	
			1 2 3 4 5	

Notes

Breakfast

Lunch

Dinner

Water 🥛🥛🥛🥛🥛🥛🥛 +

SHOW ME WHERE IT HURTS: FRONT

SHOW ME WHERE IT HURTS: BACK

MEDICATION & SUPPLIMENTS

DOSAGE	NAME	TIME

Symptom Tracker

ENERGY LEVEL

(1) (2) (3) (4) (5)

TODAY'S MOOD

WEATHER

time	symptom	trigger	severity	duration
			1 2 3 4 5	
			1 2 3 4 5	
			1 2 3 4 5	
			1 2 3 4 5	
			1 2 3 4 5	
			1 2 3 4 5	
			1 2 3 4 5	
			1 2 3 4 5	
			1 2 3 4 5	
			1 2 3 4 5	

Notes

Breakfast

Lunch

Dinner

Water

SHOW ME WHERE IT HURTS: FRONT

SHOW ME WHERE IT HURTS: BACK

MEDICATION & SUPPLIMENTS

DOSAGE	NAME	TIME

Symptom Tracker

ENERGY LEVEL

(1) (2) (3) (4) (5)

TODAY'S MOOD

WEATHER

time	symptom	trigger	severity	duration
			1 2 3 4 5	
			1 2 3 4 5	
			1 2 3 4 5	
			1 2 3 4 5	
			1 2 3 4 5	
			1 2 3 4 5	
			1 2 3 4 5	
			1 2 3 4 5	
			1 2 3 4 5	
			1 2 3 4 5	

Notes

Breakfast

Lunch

Dinner

Water 🥛🥛🥛🥛🥛🥛🥛 +

SHOW ME WHERE IT
HURTS: FRONT

SHOW ME WHERE IT
HURTS: BACK

MEDICATION
& SUPPLIMENTS

DOSAGE	NAME	TIME

Symptom Tracker

ENERGY LEVEL

(1) (2) (3) (4) (5)

TODAY'S MOOD

WEATHER

time	symptom	trigger	severity	duration
			1 2 3 4 5	
			1 2 3 4 5	
			1 2 3 4 5	
			1 2 3 4 5	
			1 2 3 4 5	
			1 2 3 4 5	
			1 2 3 4 5	
			1 2 3 4 5	
			1 2 3 4 5	
			1 2 3 4 5	

Notes

Breakfast

Lunch

Dinner

Water

SHOW ME WHERE IT HURTS: FRONT

SHOW ME WHERE IT HURTS: BACK

MEDICATION & SUPPLIMENTS

DOSAGE	NAME	TIME

Symptom Tracker

ENERGY LEVEL

(1) (2) (3) (4) (5)

TODAY'S MOOD

WEATHER

time	symptom	trigger	severity	duration
			1 2 3 4 5	
			1 2 3 4 5	
			1 2 3 4 5	
			1 2 3 4 5	
			1 2 3 4 5	
			1 2 3 4 5	
			1 2 3 4 5	
			1 2 3 4 5	
			1 2 3 4 5	
			1 2 3 4 5	

Notes

Breakfast

Lunch

Dinner

Water

SHOW ME WHERE IT HURTS: FRONT

SHOW ME WHERE IT HURTS: BACK

MEDICATION & SUPPLIMENTS

DOSAGE	NAME	TIME

Symptom Tracker

ENERGY LEVEL

(1) (2) (3) (4) (5)

TODAY'S MOOD

WEATHER

time	symptom	trigger	severity	duration
			1 2 3 4 5	
			1 2 3 4 5	
			1 2 3 4 5	
			1 2 3 4 5	
			1 2 3 4 5	
			1 2 3 4 5	
			1 2 3 4 5	
			1 2 3 4 5	
			1 2 3 4 5	
			1 2 3 4 5	

Notes

Breakfast

Lunch

Dinner

Water 🥛🥛🥛🥛🥛🥛🥛 +

SHOW ME WHERE IT
HURTS: FRONT

SHOW ME WHERE IT
HURTS: BACK

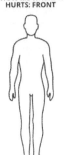

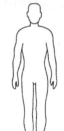

MEDICATION
& SUPPLIMENTS

DOSAGE	NAME	TIME

Symptom Tracker

ENERGY LEVEL

(1) (2) (3) (4) (5)

TODAY'S MOOD

WEATHER

time	symptom	trigger	severity	duration
			1 2 3 4 5	
			1 2 3 4 5	
			1 2 3 4 5	
			1 2 3 4 5	
			1 2 3 4 5	
			1 2 3 4 5	
			1 2 3 4 5	
			1 2 3 4 5	
			1 2 3 4 5	
			1 2 3 4 5	

Notes

Breakfast

Lunch

Dinner

Water 🥛 🥛 🥛 🥛 🥛 🥛 🥛 +

SHOW ME WHERE IT HURTS: FRONT

SHOW ME WHERE IT HURTS: BACK

MEDICATION & SUPPLIMENTS

DOSAGE	NAME	TIME

Symptom Tracker

ENERGY LEVEL   **TODAY'S MOOD**   **WEATHER**

(1) (2) (3) (4) (5)

time	symptom	trigger	severity	duration
			1 2 3 4 5	
			1 2 3 4 5	
			1 2 3 4 5	
			1 2 3 4 5	
			1 2 3 4 5	
			1 2 3 4 5	
			1 2 3 4 5	
			1 2 3 4 5	
			1 2 3 4 5	
			1 2 3 4 5	

Notes

Breakfast

Lunch

Dinner

Water   +

SHOW ME WHERE IT HURTS: FRONT   **SHOW ME WHERE IT HURTS: BACK**

MEDICATION & SUPPLIMENTS

DOSAGE	NAME	TIME

Symptom Tracker

ENERGY LEVEL

(1) (2) (3) (4) (5)

TODAY'S MOOD

WEATHER

time	symptom	trigger	severity	duration
			1 2 3 4 5	
			1 2 3 4 5	
			1 2 3 4 5	
			1 2 3 4 5	
			1 2 3 4 5	
			1 2 3 4 5	
			1 2 3 4 5	
			1 2 3 4 5	
			1 2 3 4 5	
			1 2 3 4 5	

Notes

Breakfast

Lunch

Dinner

Water ▢ ▢ ▢ ▢ ▢ ▢ ▢ +

SHOW ME WHERE IT HURTS: FRONT

SHOW ME WHERE IT HURTS: BACK

MEDICATION & SUPPLIMENTS

DOSAGE	NAME	TIME

Symptom Tracker

ENERGY LEVEL

(1) (2) (3) (4) (5)

TODAY'S MOOD

WEATHER

time	symptom	trigger	severity	duration
			1 2 3 4 5	
			1 2 3 4 5	
			1 2 3 4 5	
			1 2 3 4 5	
			1 2 3 4 5	
			1 2 3 4 5	
			1 2 3 4 5	
			1 2 3 4 5	
			1 2 3 4 5	
			1 2 3 4 5	

Notes

Breakfast

Lunch

Dinner

Water ⊔ ⊔ ⊔ ⊔ ⊔ ⊔ ⊔ +

SHOW ME WHERE IT HURTS: FRONT

SHOW ME WHERE IT HURTS: BACK

MEDICATION & SUPPLIMENTS

DOSAGE	NAME	TIME

Symptom Tracker

ENERGY LEVEL

(1) (2) (3) (4) (5)

TODAY'S MOOD

WEATHER

time	symptom	trigger	severity	duration
			1 2 3 4 5	
			1 2 3 4 5	
			1 2 3 4 5	
			1 2 3 4 5	
			1 2 3 4 5	
			1 2 3 4 5	
			1 2 3 4 5	
			1 2 3 4 5	
			1 2 3 4 5	
			1 2 3 4 5	

Notes

Breakfast

Lunch

Dinner

Water

SHOW ME WHERE IT HURTS: FRONT

SHOW ME WHERE IT HURTS: BACK

MEDICATION & SUPPLIMENTS

DOSAGE	NAME	TIME

Symptom Tracker

ENERGY LEVEL

(1) (2) (3) (4) (5)

TODAY'S MOOD

WEATHER

time	symptom	trigger	severity	duration
			1 2 3 4 5	
			1 2 3 4 5	
			1 2 3 4 5	
			1 2 3 4 5	
			1 2 3 4 5	
			1 2 3 4 5	
			1 2 3 4 5	
			1 2 3 4 5	
			1 2 3 4 5	
			1 2 3 4 5	

Notes

Breakfast

Lunch

Dinner

Water

SHOW ME WHERE IT HURTS: FRONT

SHOW ME WHERE IT HURTS: BACK

MEDICATION & SUPPLIMENTS

DOSAGE	NAME	TIME

Symptom Tracker

_____

ENERGY LEVEL   **TODAY'S MOOD**   **WEATHER**

(1) (2) (3) (4) (5)

time	symptom	trigger	severity	duration
			1 2 3 4 5	
			1 2 3 4 5	
			1 2 3 4 5	
			1 2 3 4 5	
			1 2 3 4 5	
			1 2 3 4 5	
			1 2 3 4 5	
			1 2 3 4 5	
			1 2 3 4 5	
			1 2 3 4 5	

Notes

Breakfast

Lunch

Dinner

Water

SHOW ME WHERE IT HURTS: FRONT   **SHOW ME WHERE IT HURTS: BACK**

MEDICATION & SUPPLIMENTS

DOSAGE	NAME	TIME

Symptom Tracker

ENERGY LEVEL

(1) (2) (3) (4) (5)

TODAY'S MOOD

WEATHER

time	symptom	trigger	severity	duration
			1 2 3 4 5	
			1 2 3 4 5	
			1 2 3 4 5	
			1 2 3 4 5	
			1 2 3 4 5	
			1 2 3 4 5	
			1 2 3 4 5	
			1 2 3 4 5	
			1 2 3 4 5	
			1 2 3 4 5	

Notes

Breakfast

Lunch

Dinner

Water ▢ ▢ ▢ ▢ ▢ ▢ ▢ +

SHOW ME WHERE IT HURTS: FRONT

SHOW ME WHERE IT HURTS: BACK

MEDICATION & SUPPLIMENTS

DOSAGE	NAME	TIME

Symptom Tracker

ENERGY LEVEL
(1) (2) (3) (4) (5)

TODAY'S MOOD

WEATHER

time	symptom	trigger	severity	duration
			1 2 3 4 5	
			1 2 3 4 5	
			1 2 3 4 5	
			1 2 3 4 5	
			1 2 3 4 5	
			1 2 3 4 5	
			1 2 3 4 5	
			1 2 3 4 5	
			1 2 3 4 5	
			1 2 3 4 5	

Notes

Breakfast

Lunch

Dinner

Water

SHOW ME WHERE IT HURTS: FRONT

SHOW ME WHERE IT HURTS: BACK

MEDICATION & SUPPLIMENTS

DOSAGE	NAME	TIME

Symptom Tracker

ENERGY LEVEL　　　　**TODAY'S MOOD**　　　　**WEATHER**

(1) (2) (3) (4) (5)

time	symptom	trigger	severity	duration
			1 2 3 4 5	
			1 2 3 4 5	
			1 2 3 4 5	
			1 2 3 4 5	
			1 2 3 4 5	
			1 2 3 4 5	
			1 2 3 4 5	
			1 2 3 4 5	
			1 2 3 4 5	
			1 2 3 4 5	

Notes

Breakfast

Lunch

Dinner

Water

SHOW ME WHERE IT HURTS: FRONT　　　**SHOW ME WHERE IT HURTS: BACK**

MEDICATION & SUPPLIMENTS

DOSAGE	NAME	TIME

Symptom Tracker

ENERGY LEVEL (1) (2) (3) (4) (5)

TODAY'S MOOD 😄 🙂 😐 🙁 😢

WEATHER ☀ ⛅ ☁ 🌥 🌧 ❄

time	symptom	trigger	severity	duration
			1 2 3 4 5	
			1 2 3 4 5	
			1 2 3 4 5	
			1 2 3 4 5	
			1 2 3 4 5	
			1 2 3 4 5	
			1 2 3 4 5	
			1 2 3 4 5	
			1 2 3 4 5	
			1 2 3 4 5	

Notes

Breakfast

Lunch

Dinner

Water 🥛 🥛 🥛 🥛 🥛 🥛 🥛 +

SHOW ME WHERE IT HURTS: FRONT

SHOW ME WHERE IT HURTS: BACK

MEDICATION & SUPPLIMENTS

DOSAGE	NAME	TIME

Symptom Tracker

ENERGY LEVEL

(1) (2) (3) (4) (5)

TODAY'S MOOD

WEATHER

time	symptom	trigger	severity	duration
			1 2 3 4 5	
			1 2 3 4 5	
			1 2 3 4 5	
			1 2 3 4 5	
			1 2 3 4 5	
			1 2 3 4 5	
			1 2 3 4 5	
			1 2 3 4 5	
			1 2 3 4 5	
			1 2 3 4 5	

Notes

Breakfast

Lunch

Dinner

Water 🥛🥛🥛🥛🥛🥛🥛 +

SHOW ME WHERE IT HURTS: FRONT

SHOW ME WHERE IT HURTS: BACK

MEDICATION & SUPPLIMENTS

DOSAGE	NAME	TIME

Symptom Tracker

ENERGY LEVEL

(1) (2) (3) (4) (5)

TODAY'S MOOD

WEATHER

time	symptom	trigger	severity	duration
			1 2 3 4 5	
			1 2 3 4 5	
			1 2 3 4 5	
			1 2 3 4 5	
			1 2 3 4 5	
			1 2 3 4 5	
			1 2 3 4 5	
			1 2 3 4 5	
			1 2 3 4 5	
			1 2 3 4 5	

Notes

Breakfast

Lunch

Dinner

Water □ □ □ □ □ □ □ +

SHOW ME WHERE IT HURTS: FRONT

SHOW ME WHERE IT HURTS: BACK

MEDICATION & SUPPLIMENTS

DOSAGE	NAME	TIME

Symptom Tracker

ENERGY LEVEL

(1) (2) (3) (4) (5)

TODAY'S MOOD

WEATHER

time	symptom	trigger	severity	duration
			1 2 3 4 5	
			1 2 3 4 5	
			1 2 3 4 5	
			1 2 3 4 5	
			1 2 3 4 5	
			1 2 3 4 5	
			1 2 3 4 5	
			1 2 3 4 5	
			1 2 3 4 5	
			1 2 3 4 5	

Notes

Breakfast

Lunch

Dinner

Water 🥛🥛🥛🥛🥛🥛🥛 +

SHOW ME WHERE IT HURTS: FRONT

SHOW ME WHERE IT HURTS: BACK

MEDICATION & SUPPLIMENTS

DOSAGE	NAME	TIME

Symptom Tracker

ENERGY LEVEL

(1) (2) (3) (4) (5)

TODAY'S MOOD

WEATHER

time	symptom	trigger	severity	duration
			1 2 3 4 5	
			1 2 3 4 5	
			1 2 3 4 5	
			1 2 3 4 5	
			1 2 3 4 5	
			1 2 3 4 5	
			1 2 3 4 5	
			1 2 3 4 5	
			1 2 3 4 5	
			1 2 3 4 5	

Notes

Breakfast

Lunch

Dinner

Water

SHOW ME WHERE IT HURTS: FRONT

SHOW ME WHERE IT HURTS: BACK

MEDICATION & SUPPLIMENTS

DOSAGE	NAME	TIME

Symptom Tracker

ENERGY LEVEL

(1) (2) (3) (4) (5)

TODAY'S MOOD

WEATHER

time	symptom	trigger	severity	duration
			1 2 3 4 5	
			1 2 3 4 5	
			1 2 3 4 5	
			1 2 3 4 5	
			1 2 3 4 5	
			1 2 3 4 5	
			1 2 3 4 5	
			1 2 3 4 5	
			1 2 3 4 5	
			1 2 3 4 5	

Notes

Breakfast

Lunch

Dinner

Water 🥛 🥛 🥛 🥛 🥛 🥛 🥛 +

SHOW ME WHERE IT HURTS: FRONT

SHOW ME WHERE IT HURTS: BACK

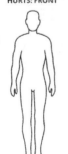

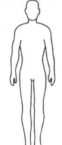

MEDICATION & SUPPLIMENTS

DOSAGE	NAME	TIME

Symptom Tracker

ENERGY LEVEL

(1) (2) (3) (4) (5)

TODAY'S MOOD

WEATHER

time	symptom	trigger	severity	duration
			1 2 3 4 5	
			1 2 3 4 5	
			1 2 3 4 5	
			1 2 3 4 5	
			1 2 3 4 5	
			1 2 3 4 5	
			1 2 3 4 5	
			1 2 3 4 5	
			1 2 3 4 5	
			1 2 3 4 5	

Notes

Breakfast

Lunch

Dinner

Water

SHOW ME WHERE IT HURTS: FRONT

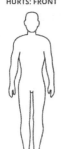

SHOW ME WHERE IT HURTS: BACK

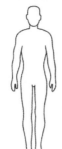

MEDICATION & SUPPLIMENTS

DOSAGE	NAME	TIME

Symptom Tracker

DATE _____

ENERGY LEVEL

① ② ③ ④ ⑤

TODAY'S MOOD

WEATHER

time	symptom	trigger	severity	duration
			1 2 3 4 5	
			1 2 3 4 5	
			1 2 3 4 5	
			1 2 3 4 5	
			1 2 3 4 5	
			1 2 3 4 5	
			1 2 3 4 5	
			1 2 3 4 5	
			1 2 3 4 5	
			1 2 3 4 5	

Notes

Breakfast

Lunch

Dinner

Water 🥛🥛🥛🥛🥛🥛🥛 +

SHOW ME WHERE IT HURTS: FRONT

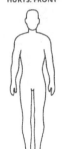

SHOW ME WHERE IT HURTS: BACK

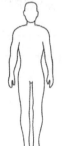

MEDICATION & SUPPLIMENTS

DOSAGE	NAME	TIME

Symptom Tracker

ENERGY LEVEL

(1) (2) (3) (4) (5)

TODAY'S MOOD

WEATHER

time	symptom	trigger	severity	duration
			1 2 3 4 5	
			1 2 3 4 5	
			1 2 3 4 5	
			1 2 3 4 5	
			1 2 3 4 5	
			1 2 3 4 5	
			1 2 3 4 5	
			1 2 3 4 5	
			1 2 3 4 5	
			1 2 3 4 5	

Notes

Breakfast

Lunch

Dinner

Water ☐ ☐ ☐ ☐ ☐ ☐ ☐ +

SHOW ME WHERE IT HURTS: FRONT

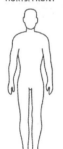

SHOW ME WHERE IT HURTS: BACK

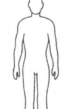

MEDICATION & SUPPLIMENTS

DOSAGE	NAME	TIME

Symptom Tracker

DATE
_____

ENERGY LEVEL

(1) (2) (0) (1) (5)

TODAY'S MOOD

WEATHER

time	symptom	trigger	severity	duration
			1 2 3 4 5	
			1 2 3 4 5	
			1 2 3 4 5	
			1 2 3 4 5	
			1 2 3 4 5	
			1 2 3 4 5	
			1 2 3 4 5	
			1 2 3 4 5	
			1 2 3 4 5	
			1 2 3 4 5	

Notes

Breakfast

Lunch

Dinner

Water 🥛 🥛 🥛 🥛 🥛 🥛 +

SHOW ME WHERE IT HURTS: FRONT

SHOW ME WHERE IT HURTS: BACK

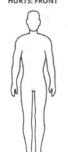

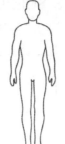

MEDICATION & SUPPLIMENTS

DOSAGE	NAME	TIME

Symptom Tracker

ENERGY LEVEL

(1) (2) (3) (4) (5)

TODAY'S MOOD

WEATHER

time	symptom	trigger	severity	duration
			1 2 3 4 5	
			1 2 3 4 5	
			1 2 3 4 5	
			1 2 3 4 5	
			1 2 3 4 5	
			1 2 3 4 5	
			1 2 3 4 5	
			1 2 3 4 5	
			1 2 3 4 5	
			1 2 3 4 5	

Notes

Breakfast

Lunch

Dinner

Water

SHOW ME WHERE IT HURTS: FRONT

SHOW ME WHERE IT HURTS: BACK

MEDICATION & SUPPLIMENTS

DOSAGE	NAME	TIME

Symptom Tracker

ENERGY LEVEL

(1) (2) (3) (4) (5)

TODAY'S MOOD

WEATHER

time	symptom	trigger	severity	duration
			1 2 3 4 5	
			1 2 3 4 5	
			1 2 3 4 5	
			1 2 3 4 5	
			1 2 3 4 5	
			1 2 3 4 5	
			1 2 3 4 5	
			1 2 3 4 5	
			1 2 3 4 5	
			1 2 3 4 5	

Notes

Breakfast

Lunch

Dinner

Water

SHOW ME WHERE IT HURTS: FRONT

SHOW ME WHERE IT HURTS: BACK

MEDICATION & SUPPLIMENTS

DOSAGE	NAME	TIME

Symptom Tracker

_____

ENERGY LEVEL

(1) (2) (3) (4) (5)

TODAY'S MOOD

WEATHER

time	symptom	trigger	severity	duration
			1 2 3 4 5	
			1 2 3 4 5	
			1 2 3 4 5	
			1 2 3 4 5	
			1 2 3 4 5	
			1 2 3 4 5	
			1 2 3 4 5	
			1 2 3 4 5	
			1 2 3 4 5	
			1 2 3 4 5	

Notes

Breakfast

Lunch

Dinner

Water 🥛 🥛 🥛 🥛 🥛 🥛 +

SHOW ME WHERE IT HURTS: FRONT

SHOW ME WHERE IT HURTS: BACK

MEDICATION & SUPPLIMENTS

DOSAGE	NAME	TIME

Symptom Tracker

ENERGY LEVEL

(1) (2) (3) (4) (5)

TODAY'S MOOD

😄 🙂 😐 🙁 😢

WEATHER

☀ ⛅ ☁ 🌦 🌧 ❄

time	symptom	trigger	severity	duration
			1 2 3 4 5	
			1 2 3 4 5	
			1 2 3 4 5	
			1 2 3 4 5	
			1 2 3 4 5	
			1 2 3 4 5	
			1 2 3 4 5	
			1 2 3 4 5	
			1 2 3 4 5	
			1 2 3 4 5	

Notes

Breakfast

Lunch

Dinner

Water 🥛 🥛 🥛 🥛 🥛 🥛 🥛 +

SHOW ME WHERE IT HURTS: FRONT

SHOW ME WHERE IT HURTS: BACK

MEDICATION & SUPPLIMENTS

DOSAGE	NAME	TIME

Symptom Tracker

ENERGY LEVEL   TODAY'S MOOD   WEATHER

(1) (2) (3) (4) (5)

time	symptom	trigger	severity	duration
			1 2 3 4 5	
			1 2 3 4 5	
			1 2 3 4 5	
			1 2 3 4 5	
			1 2 3 4 5	
			1 2 3 4 5	
			1 2 3 4 5	
			1 2 3 4 5	
			1 2 3 4 5	
			1 2 3 4 5	

Notes

Breakfast

Lunch

Dinner

Water   +

SHOW ME WHERE IT HURTS: FRONT   SHOW ME WHERE IT HURTS: BACK

MEDICATION & SUPPLIMENTS

DOSAGE	NAME	TIME

Symptom Tracker

ENERGY LEVEL

(1) (2) (3) (4) (5)

TODAY'S MOOD

WEATHER

time	symptom	trigger	severity	duration
			1 2 3 4 5	
			1 2 3 4 5	
			1 2 3 4 5	
			1 2 3 4 5	
			1 2 3 4 5	
			1 2 3 4 5	
			1 2 3 4 5	
			1 2 3 4 5	
			1 2 3 4 5	
			1 2 3 4 5	

Notes

Breakfast

Lunch

Dinner

Water 🥛 🥛 🥛 🥛 🥛 🥛 🥛 +

SHOW ME WHERE IT HURTS: FRONT

SHOW ME WHERE IT HURTS: BACK

MEDICATION & SUPPLIMENTS

DOSAGE	NAME	TIME

Symptom Tracker

ENERGY LEVEL

(1) (2) (3) (4) (5)

TODAY'S MOOD

WEATHER

time	symptom	trigger	severity	duration
			1 2 3 4 5	
			1 2 3 4 5	
			1 2 3 4 5	
			1 2 3 4 5	
			1 2 3 4 5	
			1 2 3 4 5	
			1 2 3 4 5	
			1 2 3 4 5	
			1 2 3 4 5	
			1 2 3 4 5	

Notes

Breakfast

Lunch

Dinner

Water

SHOW ME WHERE IT HURTS: FRONT

SHOW ME WHERE IT HURTS: BACK

MEDICATION & SUPPLIMENTS

DOSAGE	NAME	TIME

Symptom Tracker

ENERGY LEVEL

(1) (2) (3) (4) (5)

TODAY'S MOOD

WEATHER

time	symptom	trigger	severity	duration
			1 2 3 4 5	
			1 2 3 4 5	
			1 2 3 4 5	
			1 2 3 4 5	
			1 2 3 4 5	
			1 2 3 4 5	
			1 2 3 4 5	
			1 2 3 4 5	
			1 2 3 4 5	
			1 2 3 4 5	

Notes

Breakfast

Lunch

Dinner

Water

SHOW ME WHERE IT HURTS: FRONT

SHOW ME WHERE IT HURTS: BACK

MEDICATION & SUPPLIMENTS

DOSAGE	NAME	TIME

Symptom Tracker

ENERGY LEVEL

(1) (2) (3) (4) (5)

TODAY'S MOOD

WEATHER

time	symptom	trigger	severity	duration
			1 2 3 4 5	
			1 2 3 4 5	
			1 2 3 4 5	
			1 2 3 4 5	
			1 2 3 4 5	
			1 2 3 4 5	
			1 2 3 4 5	
			1 2 3 4 5	
			1 2 3 4 5	
			1 2 3 4 5	

Notes

Breakfast

Lunch

Dinner

Water

SHOW ME WHERE IT HURTS: FRONT

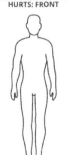

SHOW ME WHERE IT HURTS: BACK

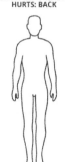

MEDICATION & SUPPLIMENTS

DOSAGE	NAME	TIME

Symptom Tracker

ENERGY LEVEL
(1) (2) (3) (4) (5)

TODAY'S MOOD

WEATHER

time	symptom	trigger	severity	duration
			1 2 3 4 5	
			1 2 3 4 5	
			1 2 3 4 5	
			1 2 3 4 5	
			1 2 3 4 5	
			1 2 3 4 5	
			1 2 3 4 5	
			1 2 3 4 5	
			1 2 3 4 5	
			1 2 3 4 5	

Notes

Breakfast

Lunch

Dinner

Water 🥛🥛🥛🥛🥛🥛🥛 +

SHOW ME WHERE IT HURTS: FRONT

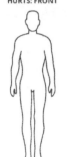

SHOW ME WHERE IT HURTS: BACK

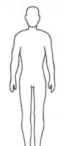

MEDICATION & SUPPLIMENTS

DOSAGE	NAME	TIME

Symptom Tracker

ENERGY LEVEL

(1) (2) (3) (4) (5)

TODAY'S MOOD

WEATHER

time	symptom	trigger	severity	duration
			1 2 3 4 5	
			1 2 3 4 5	
			1 2 3 4 5	
			1 2 3 4 5	
			1 2 3 4 5	
			1 2 3 4 5	
			1 2 3 4 5	
			1 2 3 4 5	
			1 2 3 4 5	
			1 2 3 4 5	

Notes

Breakfast

Lunch

Dinner

Water ▽ ▽ ▽ ▽ ▽ ▽ ▽ +

SHOW ME WHERE IT HURTS: FRONT

SHOW ME WHERE IT HURTS: BACK

MEDICATION & SUPPLIMENTS

DOSAGE	NAME	TIME

Symptom Tracker

ENERGY LEVEL　　　　　**TODAY'S MOOD**　　　　　**WEATHER**

(1)　(2)　(3)　(4)　(5)

time	symptom	trigger	severity	duration
			1 2 3 4 5	
			1 2 3 4 5	
			1 2 3 4 5	
			1 2 3 4 5	
			1 2 3 4 5	
			1 2 3 4 5	
			1 2 3 4 5	
			1 2 3 4 5	
			1 2 3 4 5	
			1 2 3 4 5	

Notes

Breakfast

Lunch

Dinner

Water ⎕ ⎕ ⎕ ⎕ ⎕ ⎕ ⎕ +

SHOW ME WHERE IT HURTS: FRONT　　**SHOW ME WHERE IT HURTS: BACK**

MEDICATION & SUPPLIMENTS

DOSAGE	NAME	TIME

Symptom Tracker

ENERGY LEVEL

(1) (2) (3) (4) (5)

TODAY'S MOOD

WEATHER

time	symptom	trigger	severity	duration
			1 2 3 4 5	
			1 2 3 4 5	
			1 2 3 4 5	
			1 2 3 4 5	
			1 2 3 4 5	
			1 2 3 4 5	
			1 2 3 4 5	
			1 2 3 4 5	
			1 2 3 4 5	
			1 2 3 4 5	

Notes

Breakfast

Lunch

Dinner

Water 🥛 🥛 🥛 🥛 🥛 🥛 +

SHOW ME WHERE IT HURTS: FRONT

SHOW ME WHERE IT HURTS: BACK

MEDICATION & SUPPLIMENTS

DOSAGE	NAME	TIME

Symptom Tracker

ENERGY LEVEL

(1) (2) (3) (4) (5)

TODAY'S MOOD

WEATHER

time	symptom	trigger	severity	duration
			1 2 3 4 5	
			1 2 3 4 5	
			1 2 3 4 5	
			1 2 3 4 5	
			1 2 3 4 5	
			1 2 3 4 5	
			1 2 3 4 5	
			1 2 3 4 5	
			1 2 3 4 5	
			1 2 3 4 5	

Notes

Breakfast

Lunch

Dinner

Water

**SHOW ME WHERE IT
HURTS: FRONT**

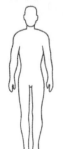

**SHOW ME WHERE IT
HURTS: BACK**

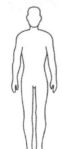

MEDICATION
& SUPPLIMENTS

DOSAGE	NAME	TIME

Symptom Tracker

ENERGY LEVEL

(1) (2) (3) (4) (5)

TODAY'S MOOD

WEATHER

time	symptom	trigger	severity	duration
			1 2 3 4 5	
			1 2 3 4 5	
			1 2 3 4 5	
			1 2 3 4 5	
			1 2 3 4 5	
			1 2 3 4 5	
			1 2 3 4 5	
			1 2 3 4 5	
			1 2 3 4 5	
			1 2 3 4 5	

Notes

Breakfast

Lunch

Dinner

Water +

SHOW ME WHERE IT HURTS: FRONT

SHOW ME WHERE IT HURTS: BACK

MEDICATION & SUPPLIMENTS

DOSAGE	NAME	TIME

Symptom Tracker

ENERGY LEVEL

(1) (2) (3) (4) (5)

TODAY'S MOOD

WEATHER

time	symptom	trigger	severity	duration
			1 2 3 4 5	
			1 2 3 4 5	
			1 2 3 4 5	
			1 2 3 4 5	
			1 2 3 4 5	
			1 2 3 4 5	
			1 2 3 4 5	
			1 2 3 4 5	
			1 2 3 4 5	
			1 2 3 4 5	

Notes

Breakfast

Lunch

Dinner

Water 🥛🥛🥛🥛🥛🥛🥛 +

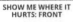
SHOW ME WHERE IT HURTS: FRONT

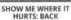
SHOW ME WHERE IT HURTS: BACK

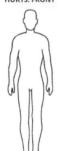

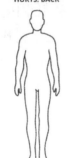

MEDICATION & SUPPLIMENTS

DOSAGE	NAME	TIME

Symptom Tracker

ENERGY LEVEL

(1) (2) (3) (4) (5)

TODAY'S MOOD

WEATHER

time	symptom	trigger	severity	duration
			1 2 3 4 5	
			1 2 3 4 5	
			1 2 3 4 5	
			1 2 3 4 5	
			1 2 3 4 5	
			1 2 3 4 5	
			1 2 3 4 5	
			1 2 3 4 5	
			1 2 3 4 5	
			1 2 3 4 5	

Notes

Breakfast

Lunch

Dinner

Water +

SHOW ME WHERE IT HURTS: FRONT

SHOW ME WHERE IT HURTS: BACK

MEDICATION & SUPPLIMENTS

DOSAGE	NAME	TIME

Symptom Tracker

ENERGY LEVEL

(1) (2) (3) (4) (5)

TODAY'S MOOD

WEATHER

time	symptom	trigger	severity	duration
			1 2 3 4 5	
			1 2 3 4 5	
			1 2 3 4 5	
			1 2 3 4 5	
			1 2 3 4 5	
			1 2 3 4 5	
			1 2 3 4 5	
			1 2 3 4 5	
			1 2 3 4 5	
			1 2 3 4 5	

Notes

Breakfast

Lunch

Dinner

Water 🥛 🥛 🥛 🥛 🥛 🥛 🥛 +

SHOW ME WHERE IT HURTS: FRONT

SHOW ME WHERE IT HURTS: BACK

MEDICATION & SUPPLIMENTS

DOSAGE	NAME	TIME

Symptom Tracker

ENERGY LEVEL

(1) (2) (3) (4) (5)

TODAY'S MOOD

😄 🙂 😐 🙁 😣

WEATHER

☀ ⛅ ☁ 🌬 🌧 ❄

time	symptom	trigger	severity	duration
			1 2 3 4 5	
			1 2 3 4 5	
			1 2 3 4 5	
			1 2 3 4 5	
			1 2 3 4 5	
			1 2 3 4 5	
			1 2 3 4 5	
			1 2 3 4 5	
			1 2 3 4 5	
			1 2 3 4 5	

Notes

Breakfast

Lunch

Dinner

Water 🥛 🥛 🥛 🥛 🥛 🥛 +

SHOW ME WHERE IT HURTS: FRONT

SHOW ME WHERE IT HURTS: BACK

MEDICATION & SUPPLIMENTS

DOSAGE	NAME	TIME

Symptom Tracker

ENERGY LEVEL

(1) (2) (3) (4) (5)

TODAY'S MOOD

WEATHER

time	symptom	trigger	severity	duration
			1 2 3 4 5	
			1 2 3 4 5	
			1 2 3 4 5	
			1 2 3 4 5	
			1 2 3 4 5	
			1 2 3 4 5	
			1 2 3 4 5	
			1 2 3 4 5	
			1 2 3 4 5	
			1 2 3 4 5	

Notes

Breakfast

Lunch

Dinner

Water +

SHOW ME WHERE IT HURTS: FRONT

SHOW ME WHERE IT HURTS: BACK

MEDICATION & SUPPLIMENTS

DOSAGE	NAME	TIME

Symptom Tracker

ENERGY LEVEL

(1)　(2)　(3)　(4)　(5)

TODAY'S MOOD

WEATHER

time	symptom	trigger	severity	duration
			1 2 3 4 5	
			1 2 3 4 5	
			1 2 3 4 5	
			1 2 3 4 5	
			1 2 3 4 5	
			1 2 3 4 5	
			1 2 3 4 5	
			1 2 3 4 5	
			1 2 3 4 5	
			1 2 3 4 5	

Notes

Breakfast

Lunch

Dinner

Water ▢ ▢ ▢ ▢ ▢ ▢ ▢ +

SHOW ME WHERE IT HURTS: FRONT

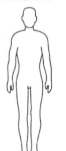

SHOW ME WHERE IT HURTS: BACK

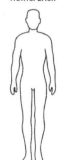

MEDICATION & SUPPLIMENTS

DOSAGE	NAME	TIME

Symptom Tracker

ENERGY LEVEL
(1) (2) (3) (4) (5)

TODAY'S MOOD
😄 🙂 😐 🙁 😢

WEATHER
☀️ 🌤️ ☁️ 🌧️ ⛈️ ❄️

time	symptom	trigger	severity	duration
			1 2 3 4 5	
			1 2 3 4 5	
			1 2 3 4 5	
			1 2 3 4 5	
			1 2 3 4 5	
			1 2 3 4 5	
			1 2 3 4 5	
			1 2 3 4 5	
			1 2 3 4 5	
			1 2 3 4 5	

Notes

Breakfast

Lunch

Dinner

Water 🥛 🥛 🥛 🥛 🥛 🥛 🥛 +

SHOW ME WHERE IT HURTS: FRONT

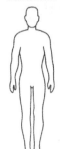

SHOW ME WHERE IT HURTS: BACK

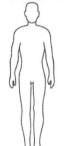

MEDICATION & SUPPLIMENTS

DOSAGE	NAME	TIME

Symptom Tracker

ENERGY LEVEL

(1) (2) (3) (4) (5)

TODAY'S MOOD

WEATHER

time	symptom	trigger	severity	duration
			1 2 3 4 5	
			1 2 3 4 5	
			1 2 3 4 5	
			1 2 3 4 5	
			1 2 3 4 5	
			1 2 3 4 5	
			1 2 3 4 5	
			1 2 3 4 5	
			1 2 3 4 5	
			1 2 3 4 5	

Notes

Breakfast

Lunch

Dinner

Water

SHOW ME WHERE IT
HURTS: FRONT

SHOW ME WHERE IT
HURTS: BACK

MEDICATION & SUPPLIMENTS

DOSAGE	NAME	TIME

Symptom Tracker

ENERGY LEVEL

(1) (2) (3) (4) (5)

TODAY'S MOOD

WEATHER

time	symptom	trigger	severity	duration
			1 2 3 4 5	
			1 2 3 4 5	
			1 2 3 4 5	
			1 2 3 4 5	
			1 2 3 4 5	
			1 2 3 4 5	
			1 2 3 4 5	
			1 2 3 4 5	
			1 2 3 4 5	
			1 2 3 4 5	

Notes

Breakfast

Lunch

Dinner

Water +

SHOW ME WHERE IT HURTS: FRONT

SHOW ME WHERE IT HURTS: BACK

MEDICATION & SUPPLIMENTS

DOSAGE	NAME	TIME

Symptom Tracker

ENERGY LEVEL

(1) (2) (3) (4) (5)

TODAY'S MOOD

WEATHER

time	symptom	trigger	severity	duration
			1 2 3 4 5	
			1 2 3 4 5	
			1 2 3 4 5	
			1 2 3 4 5	
			1 2 3 4 5	
			1 2 3 4 5	
			1 2 3 4 5	
			1 2 3 4 5	
			1 2 3 4 5	
			1 2 3 4 5	

Notes

Breakfast

Lunch

Dinner

Water ⛾ ⛾ ⛾ ⛾ ⛾ ⛾ +

SHOW ME WHERE IT HURTS: FRONT

SHOW ME WHERE IT HURTS: BACK

MEDICATION & SUPPLIMENTS

DOSAGE	NAME	TIME

Symptom Tracker

ENERGY LEVEL
(1) (2) (3) (4) (5)

TODAY'S MOOD
😌 🙂 😐 🙁 😞

WEATHER
☀ ⛅ ☁ 🌧 🌧 ❄

time	symptom	trigger	severity	duration
			1 2 3 4 5	
			1 2 3 4 5	
			1 2 3 4 5	
			1 2 3 4 5	
			1 2 3 4 5	
			1 2 3 4 5	
			1 2 3 4 5	
			1 2 3 4 5	
			1 2 3 4 5	
			1 2 3 4 5	

Notes

Breakfast

Lunch

Dinner

Water 🥛🥛🥛🥛🥛🥛🥛 +

SHOW ME WHERE IT HURTS: FRONT

SHOW ME WHERE IT HURTS: BACK

MEDICATION & SUPPLIMENTS

DOSAGE	NAME	TIME

Symptom Tracker

ENERGY LEVEL

(1) (2) (3) (4) (5)

TODAY'S MOOD

WEATHER

time	symptom	trigger	severity	duration
			1 2 3 4 5	
			1 2 3 4 5	
			1 2 3 4 5	
			1 2 3 4 5	
			1 2 3 4 5	
			1 2 3 4 5	
			1 2 3 4 5	
			1 2 3 4 5	
			1 2 3 4 5	
			1 2 3 4 5	

Notes

Breakfast

Lunch

Dinner

Water 🥛 🥛 🥛 🥛 🥛 🥛 🥛 +

SHOW ME WHERE IT HURTS: FRONT

SHOW ME WHERE IT HURTS: BACK

MEDICATION & SUPPLIMENTS

DOSAGE	NAME	TIME

Symptom Tracker

ENERGY LEVEL

(1) (2) (3) (4) (5)

TODAY'S MOOD

WEATHER

time	symptom	trigger	severity	duration
			1 2 3 4 5	
			1 2 3 4 5	
			1 2 3 4 5	
			1 2 3 4 5	
			1 2 3 4 5	
			1 2 3 4 5	
			1 2 3 4 5	
			1 2 3 4 5	
			1 2 3 4 5	
			1 2 3 4 5	

Notes

Breakfast

Lunch

Dinner

Water ☐ ☐ ☐ ☐ ☐ ☐ ☐ +

SHOW ME WHERE IT HURTS: FRONT

SHOW ME WHERE IT HURTS: BACK

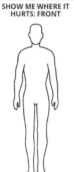

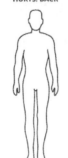

MEDICATION & SUPPLIMENTS

DOSAGE	NAME	TIME

Symptom Tracker

ENERGY LEVEL   TODAY'S MOOD   WEATHER

(1) (2) (3) (4) (5)

time	symptom	trigger	severity	duration
			1 2 3 4 5	
			1 2 3 4 5	
			1 2 3 4 5	
			1 2 3 4 5	
			1 2 3 4 5	
			1 2 3 4 5	
			1 2 3 4 5	
			1 2 3 4 5	
			1 2 3 4 5	
			1 2 3 4 5	

Notes

Breakfast

Lunch

Dinner

Water +

SHOW ME WHERE IT HURTS: FRONT   SHOW ME WHERE IT HURTS: BACK

MEDICATION & SUPPLIMENTS

DOSAGE	NAME	TIME

Symptom Tracker

ENERGY LEVEL
(1) (2) (3) (4) (5)

TODAY'S MOOD

WEATHER

time	symptom	trigger	severity	duration
			1 2 3 4 5	
			1 2 3 4 5	
			1 2 3 4 5	
			1 2 3 4 5	
			1 2 3 4 5	
			1 2 3 4 5	
			1 2 3 4 5	
			1 2 3 4 5	
			1 2 3 4 5	
			1 2 3 4 5	

Notes

Breakfast

Lunch

Dinner

Water ▯ ▯ ▯ ▯ ▯ ▯ ▯ +

SHOW ME WHERE IT HURTS: FRONT

SHOW ME WHERE IT HURTS: BACK

MEDICATION & SUPPLIMENTS

DOSAGE	NAME	TIME

Symptom Tracker

ENERGY LEVEL

(1) (2) (3) (4) (5)

TODAY'S MOOD

WEATHER

time	symptom	trigger	severity	duration
			1 2 3 4 5	
			1 2 3 4 5	
			1 2 3 4 5	
			1 2 3 4 5	
			1 2 3 4 5	
			1 2 3 4 5	
			1 2 3 4 5	
			1 2 3 4 5	
			1 2 3 4 5	
			1 2 3 4 5	

Notes

Breakfast

Lunch

Dinner

Water ☐ ☐ ☐ ☐ ☐ ☐ +

SHOW ME WHERE IT HURTS: FRONT

SHOW ME WHERE IT HURTS: BACK

MEDICATION & SUPPLIMENTS

DOSAGE	NAME	TIME

Symptom Tracker

ENERGY LEVEL

(1)(2)(3)(4)(5)

TODAY'S MOOD

WEATHER

time	symptom	trigger	severity	duration
			1 2 3 4 5	
			1 2 3 4 5	
			1 2 3 4 5	
			1 2 3 4 5	
			1 2 3 4 5	
			1 2 3 4 5	
			1 2 3 4 5	
			1 2 3 4 5	
			1 2 3 4 5	
			1 2 3 4 5	

Notes

Breakfast

Lunch

Dinner

Water +

SHOW ME WHERE IT HURTS: FRONT

SHOW ME WHERE IT HURTS: BACK

MEDICATION & SUPPLIMENTS

DOSAGE	NAME	TIME

Symptom Tracker

ENERGY LEVEL

(1) (2) (3) (4) (5)

TODAY'S MOOD

WEATHER

time	symptom	trigger	severity	duration
			1 2 3 4 5	
			1 2 3 4 5	
			1 2 3 4 5	
			1 2 3 4 5	
			1 2 3 4 5	
			1 2 3 4 5	
			1 2 3 4 5	
			1 2 3 4 5	
			1 2 3 4 5	
			1 2 3 4 5	

Notes

Breakfast

Lunch

Dinner

Water

SHOW ME WHERE IT HURTS: FRONT

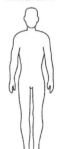

SHOW ME WHERE IT HURTS: BACK

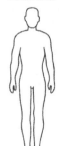

MEDICATION & SUPPLIMENTS

DOSAGE	NAME	TIME

Symptom Tracker

ENERGY LEVEL

(1)(2)(3)(4)(5)

TODAY'S MOOD

WEATHER

time	symptom	trigger	severity	duration
			1 2 3 4 5	
			1 2 3 4 5	
			1 2 3 4 5	
			1 2 3 4 5	
			1 2 3 4 5	
			1 2 3 4 5	
			1 2 3 4 5	
			1 2 3 4 5	
			1 2 3 4 5	
			1 2 3 4 5	

Notes

Breakfast

Lunch

Dinner

Water +

SHOW ME WHERE IT HURTS: FRONT

SHOW ME WHERE IT HURTS: BACK

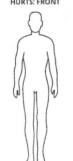

MEDICATION & SUPPLIMENTS

DOSAGE	NAME	TIME

Symptom Tracker

ENERGY LEVEL

(1) (2) (3) (4) (5)

TODAY'S MOOD

WEATHER

time	symptom	trigger	severity	duration
			1 2 3 4 5	
			1 2 3 4 5	
			1 2 3 4 5	
			1 2 3 4 5	
			1 2 3 4 5	
			1 2 3 4 5	
			1 2 3 4 5	
			1 2 3 4 5	
			1 2 3 4 5	
			1 2 3 4 5	

Notes

Breakfast

Lunch

Dinner

Water ▯ ▯ ▯ ▯ ▯ ▯ ▯ +

SHOW ME WHERE IT HURTS: FRONT

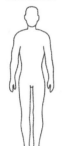

SHOW ME WHERE IT HURTS: BACK

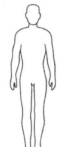

MEDICATION & SUPPLIMENTS

DOSAGE	NAME	TIME

Symptom Tracker

ENERGY LEVEL

(1) (2) (3) (4) (5)

TODAY'S MOOD

WEATHER

time	symptom	trigger	severity	duration
			1 2 3 4 5	
			1 2 3 4 5	
			1 2 3 4 5	
			1 2 3 4 5	
			1 2 3 4 5	
			1 2 3 4 5	
			1 2 3 4 5	
			1 2 3 4 5	
			1 2 3 4 5	
			1 2 3 4 5	

Notes

Breakfast

Lunch

Dinner

Water 🥛🥛🥛🥛🥛🥛 +

SHOW ME WHERE IT HURTS: FRONT

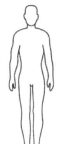

SHOW ME WHERE IT HURTS: BACK

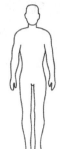

MEDICATION & SUPPLIMENTS

DOSAGE	NAME	TIME

Symptom Tracker

ENERGY LEVEL

(1) (2) (3) (4) (5)

TODAY'S MOOD

WEATHER

time	symptom	trigger	severity	duration
			1 2 3 4 5	
			1 2 3 4 5	
			1 2 3 4 5	
			1 2 3 4 5	
			1 2 3 4 5	
			1 2 3 4 5	
			1 2 3 4 5	
			1 2 3 4 5	
			1 2 3 4 5	
			1 2 3 4 5	

Notes

Breakfast

Lunch

Dinner

Water

SHOW ME WHERE IT HURTS: FRONT

SHOW ME WHERE IT HURTS: BACK

MEDICATION & SUPPLIMENTS

DOSAGE	NAME	TIME

Symptom Tracker

ENERGY LEVEL

(1) (2) (3) (4) (5)

TODAY'S MOOD

WEATHER

time	symptom	trigger	severity	duration
			1 2 3 4 5	
			1 2 3 4 5	
			1 2 3 4 5	
			1 2 3 4 5	
			1 2 3 4 5	
			1 2 3 4 5	
			1 2 3 4 5	
			1 2 3 4 5	
			1 2 3 4 5	
			1 2 3 4 5	

Notes

Breakfast

Lunch

Dinner

Water 🥛🥛🥛🥛🥛🥛🥛 +

SHOW ME WHERE IT HURTS: FRONT

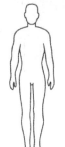

SHOW ME WHERE IT HURTS: BACK

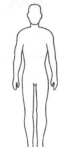

MEDICATION & SUPPLIMENTS

DOSAGE	NAME	TIME

Symptom Tracker

ENERGY LEVEL

(1) (2) (3) (4) (5)

TODAY'S MOOD

WEATHER

time	symptom	trigger	severity	duration
			1 2 3 4 5	
			1 2 3 4 5	
			1 2 3 4 5	
			1 2 3 4 5	
			1 2 3 4 5	
			1 2 3 4 5	
			1 2 3 4 5	
			1 2 3 4 5	
			1 2 3 4 5	
			1 2 3 4 5	

Notes

Breakfast

Lunch

Dinner

Water ▯ ▯ ▯ ▯ ▯ ▯ ▯ +

SHOW ME WHERE IT HURTS: FRONT

SHOW ME WHERE IT HURTS: BACK

MEDICATION & SUPPLIMENTS

DOSAGE	NAME	TIME

Symptom Tracker

ENERGY LEVEL

(1) (2) (3) (4) (5)

TODAY'S MOOD

😀 🙂 😐 🙁 😟

WEATHER

☀️ ⛅ ☁️ 🌬️ 🌧️ ❄️

time	symptom	trigger	severity	duration
			1 2 3 4 5	
			1 2 3 4 5	
			1 2 3 4 5	
			1 2 3 4 5	
			1 2 3 4 5	
			1 2 3 4 5	
			1 2 3 4 5	
			1 2 3 4 5	
			1 2 3 4 5	
			1 2 3 4 5	

Notes

Breakfast

Lunch

Dinner

Water 🥛 🥛 🥛 🥛 🥛 🥛 +

SHOW ME WHERE IT HURTS: FRONT

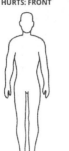

SHOW ME WHERE IT HURTS: BACK

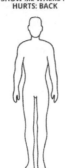

MEDICATION & SUPPLIMENTS

DOSAGE	NAME	TIME

Symptom Tracker

ENERGY LEVEL

(1) (2) (3) (4) (5)

TODAY'S MOOD

WEATHER

time	symptom	trigger	severity	duration
			1 2 3 4 5	
			1 2 3 4 5	
			1 2 3 4 5	
			1 2 3 4 5	
			1 2 3 4 5	
			1 2 3 4 5	
			1 2 3 4 5	
			1 2 3 4 5	
			1 2 3 4 5	
			1 2 3 4 5	

Notes

Breakfast

Lunch

Dinner

Water

SHOW ME WHERE IT HURTS: FRONT

SHOW ME WHERE IT HURTS: BACK

MEDICATION & SUPPLIMENTS

DOSAGE	NAME	TIME

Symptom Tracker

ENERGY LEVEL

(1) (2) (3) (4) (5)

TODAY'S MOOD

WEATHER

time	symptom	trigger	severity	duration
			1 2 3 4 5	
			1 2 3 4 5	
			1 2 3 4 5	
			1 2 3 4 5	
			1 2 3 4 5	
			1 2 3 4 5	
			1 2 3 4 5	
			1 2 3 4 5	
			1 2 3 4 5	
			1 2 3 4 5	

Notes

Breakfast

Lunch

Dinner

Water

SHOW ME WHERE IT HURTS: FRONT

SHOW ME WHERE IT HURTS: BACK

MEDICATION & SUPPLIMENTS

DOSAGE	NAME	TIME

Symptom Tracker

_____

ENERGY LEVEL   **TODAY'S MOOD**   **WEATHER**

(1) (2) (3) (4) (5)

time	symptom	trigger	severity	duration
			1 2 3 4 5	
			1 2 3 4 5	
			1 2 3 4 5	
			1 2 3 4 5	
			1 2 3 4 5	
			1 2 3 4 5	
			1 2 3 4 5	
			1 2 3 4 5	
			1 2 3 4 5	
			1 2 3 4 5	

Notes

Breakfast

Lunch

Dinner

Water 🥛🥛🥛🥛🥛🥛 +

SHOW ME WHERE IT HURTS: FRONT   **SHOW ME WHERE IT HURTS: BACK**

MEDICATION & SUPPLIMENTS

DOSAGE	NAME	TIME

Symptom Tracker

ENERGY LEVEL

(1) (2) (3) (4) (5)

TODAY'S MOOD

WEATHER

time	symptom	trigger	severity	duration
			1 2 3 4 5	
			1 2 3 4 5	
			1 2 3 4 5	
			1 2 3 4 5	
			1 2 3 4 5	
			1 2 3 4 5	
			1 2 3 4 5	
			1 2 3 4 5	
			1 2 3 4 5	
			1 2 3 4 5	

Notes

Breakfast

Lunch

Dinner

Water +

SHOW ME WHERE IT HURTS: FRONT

SHOW ME WHERE IT HURTS: BACK

MEDICATION & SUPPLIMENTS

DOSAGE	NAME	TIME

Symptom Tracker

ENERGY LEVEL

(1) (2) (3) (4) (5)

TODAY'S MOOD

WEATHER

time	symptom	trigger	severity	duration
			1 2 3 4 5	
			1 2 3 4 5	
			1 2 3 4 5	
			1 2 3 4 5	
			1 2 3 4 5	
			1 2 3 4 5	
			1 2 3 4 5	
			1 2 3 4 5	
			1 2 3 4 5	
			1 2 3 4 5	

Notes

Breakfast

Lunch

Dinner

Water

SHOW ME WHERE IT HURTS: FRONT

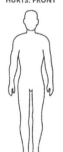

SHOW ME WHERE IT HURTS: BACK

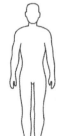

MEDICATION & SUPPLIMENTS

DOSAGE	NAME	TIME

Symptom Tracker

ENERGY LEVEL
(1) (2) (3) (4) (5)

TODAY'S MOOD
😄 🙂 😐 🙁 😢

WEATHER
☀ ⛅ ☁ 🌬 🌧 ❄

time	symptom	trigger	severity	duration
			1 2 3 4 5	
			1 2 3 4 5	
			1 2 3 4 5	
			1 2 3 4 5	
			1 2 3 4 5	
			1 2 3 4 5	
			1 2 3 4 5	
			1 2 3 4 5	
			1 2 3 4 5	
			1 2 3 4 5	

Notes

Breakfast

Lunch

Dinner

Water 🥛🥛🥛🥛🥛🥛🥛 +

SHOW ME WHERE IT HURTS: FRONT

SHOW ME WHERE IT HURTS: BACK

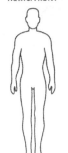
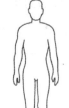

MEDICATION & SUPPLIMENTS

DOSAGE	NAME	TIME

Symptom Tracker

ENERGY LEVEL   **TODAY'S MOOD**   **WEATHER**

(1) (2) (3) (4) (5)

time	symptom	trigger	severity	duration
			1 2 3 4 5	
			1 2 3 4 5	
			1 2 3 4 5	
			1 2 3 4 5	
			1 2 3 4 5	
			1 2 3 4 5	
			1 2 3 4 5	
			1 2 3 4 5	
			1 2 3 4 5	
			1 2 3 4 5	

Notes

Breakfast

Lunch

Dinner

Water   ☐ ☐ ☐ ☐ ☐ ☐ ☐ +

SHOW ME WHERE IT HURTS: FRONT   **SHOW ME WHERE IT HURTS: BACK**

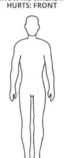
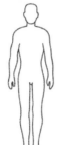

MEDICATION & SUPPLIMENTS

DOSAGE	NAME	TIME

Symptom Tracker

ENERGY LEVEL

(1) (2) (3) (4) (5)

TODAY'S MOOD

WEATHER

time	symptom	trigger	severity	duration
			1 2 3 4 5	
			1 2 3 4 5	
			1 2 3 4 5	
			1 2 3 4 5	
			1 2 3 4 5	
			1 2 3 4 5	
			1 2 3 4 5	
			1 2 3 4 5	
			1 2 3 4 5	
			1 2 3 4 5	

Notes

Breakfast

Lunch

Dinner

Water

SHOW ME WHERE IT HURTS: FRONT

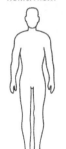

SHOW ME WHERE IT HURTS: BACK

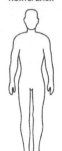

MEDICATION & SUPPLIMENTS

DOSAGE	NAME	TIME

Symptom Tracker

ENERGY LEVEL

(1) (2) (3) (4) (5)

TODAY'S MOOD

WEATHER

time	symptom	trigger	severity	duration
			1 2 3 4 5	
			1 2 3 4 5	
			1 2 3 4 5	
			1 2 3 4 5	
			1 2 3 4 5	
			1 2 3 4 5	
			1 2 3 4 5	
			1 2 3 4 5	
			1 2 3 4 5	
			1 2 3 4 5	

Notes

Breakfast

Lunch

Dinner

Water

SHOW ME WHERE IT HURTS: FRONT

SHOW ME WHERE IT HURTS: BACK

MEDICATION & SUPPLIMENTS

DOSAGE	NAME	TIME

Symptom Tracker

ENERGY LEVEL

(1) (2) (3) (4) (5)

TODAY'S MOOD

WEATHER

time	symptom	trigger	severity	duration
			1 2 3 4 5	
			1 2 3 4 5	
			1 2 3 4 5	
			1 2 3 4 5	
			1 2 3 4 5	
			1 2 3 4 5	
			1 2 3 4 5	
			1 2 3 4 5	
			1 2 3 4 5	
			1 2 3 4 5	

Notes

Breakfast

Lunch

Dinner

Water ▯ ▯ ▯ ▯ ▯ ▯ ▯ +

SHOW ME WHERE IT HURTS: FRONT

SHOW ME WHERE IT HURTS: BACK

MEDICATION & SUPPLIMENTS

DOSAGE	NAME	TIME

Appointment Checklist

Week Before
- Confirm appointment
- Confirm time, date & address
- Double-check what you need to take
- Check if you'll need to fast

Day Before
- Write down all medications & doses
- Figure out a route to the office
- Make sure to have any paperwork/test results/referral papers
- Confirm ride/transportation
- Put all paperwork in easy to find location
- Fast if necessary

Morning Of
- Choose appropriate outfit
- Double-check paperwork
- Double check route and timing
- Take snack if fasting
- Take bottle of water
- Gather bottles of medications if necessary

NOTES

Appointment Checklist

Other Care Partners	<ul><li>Pharmacist</li><li>Chiropractor</li><li>Physical therapist</li><li>Naturopath</li><li>Dentist</li></ul>
Regular Maintenence	<ul><li>FAMILY DOCTOR annual checkup & flu shots</li><li>PEDIATRICIAN annual checkups for kids</li><li>GYNECOLOGIST annual checkups for women</li><li>DERMATOLOGIST annual skin care checkup</li><li>DENTIST bi-annual checkups</li><li>EYE CARE DOCTOR every few years as needed for prescriptions & concerns</li></ul>
New Patient Checklist	<ul><li>Photo Id</li><li>Insurance cards</li><li>List of all medications</li><li>Medical records</li><li>Pharmacy name and address</li><li>Any forms required by doctor's office</li></ul>

NOTES

Appointment Notes

DATE_____   **DOCTOR**_____

Reason for
appointment

_____
_____
_____
_____
_____

Questions to
ask the
doctor

_____
_____
_____
_____
_____

Notes

_____
_____
_____
_____

NEXT APPOINTMENT _____

Appointment Notes

DATE_____   **DOCTOR**_____

Reason for
appointment

_____
_____
_____
_____
_____

Questions to
ask the
doctor

_____
_____
_____
_____
_____

Notes

_____
_____
_____
_____

NEXT APPOINTMENT _____

Appointment Notes

DATE _____   **DOCTOR** _____

Reason for
appointment

_____
_____
_____
_____
_____

Questions to
ask the
doctor

_____
_____
_____
_____
_____
_____

Notes

_____
_____
_____
_____

NEXT APPOINTMENT _____

Appointment Notes

DATE_____   **DOCTOR**_____

Reason for
appointment
_____
_____
_____
_____
_____
_____

Questions to
ask the
doctor
_____
_____
_____
_____
_____
_____

Notes
_____
_____
_____
_____
_____

NEXT APPOINTMENT _____

Appointment Notes

DATE_____   **DOCTOR**_____

Reason for
appointment

_____
_____
_____
_____
_____

Questions to
ask the
doctor

_____
_____
_____
_____
_____
_____

Notes

_____
_____
_____
_____

NEXT APPOINTMENT _____

Appointment Notes

DATE_____ **DOCTOR**_____

Reason for
appointment

_____
_____
_____
_____
_____

Questions to
ask the
doctor

_____
_____
_____
_____
_____
_____

Notes

_____
_____
_____
_____

NEXT APPOINTMENT _____

Appointment Notes

DATE _____   **DOCTOR** _____

Reason for
appointment
_____
_____
_____
_____
_____
_____

Questions to
ask the
doctor
_____
_____
_____
_____
_____
_____

Notes
_____
_____
_____
_____

NEXT APPOINTMENT _____

Appointment Notes

DATE_____   **DOCTOR**_____

Reason for
appointment
_____
_____
_____
_____
_____
_____

Questions to
ask the
doctor
_____
_____
_____
_____
_____
_____

Notes
_____
_____
_____
_____

NEXT APPOINTMENT _____

Appointment Notes

DATE_____   **DOCTOR**_____

Reason for
appointment

_____
_____
_____
_____
_____

Questions to
ask the
doctor

_____
_____
_____
_____
_____
_____

Notes

_____
_____
_____
_____

NEXT APPOINTMENT _____

Appointment Notes

DATE_____   **DOCTOR**_____

Reason for
appointment
_____
_____
_____
_____
_____

Questions to
ask the
doctor
_____
_____
_____
_____
_____
_____

Notes
_____
_____
_____
_____
_____

NEXT APPOINTMENT _____

Appointment Notes

DATE_____   DOCTOR _____

Reason for
appointment
_____
_____
_____
_____
_____

Questions to
ask the
doctor
_____
_____
_____
_____
_____

Notes
_____
_____
_____
_____

NEXT APPOINTMENT _____

Appointment Notes

DATE_____ **DOCTOR**_____

Reason for
appointment
_____
_____
_____
_____
_____

Questions to
ask the
doctor
_____
_____
_____
_____
_____
_____

Notes
_____
_____
_____
_____

NEXT APPOINTMENT _____

Appointment Notes

DATE_____   **DOCTOR**_____

Reason for
appointment

_____

_____

_____

_____

_____

Questions to
ask the
doctor

_____

_____

_____

_____

_____

_____

Notes

_____

_____

_____

_____

NEXT APPOINTMENT _____

Appointment Notes

DATE_____ **DOCTOR**_____

Reason for
appointment
_____
_____
_____
_____
_____
_____

Questions to
ask the
doctor
_____
_____
_____
_____
_____
_____

Notes
_____
_____
_____
_____
_____

NEXT APPOINTMENT _____

Appointment Notes

DATE_____ **DOCTOR**_____

Reason for
appointment

Questions to
ask the
doctor

Notes

NEXT APPOINTMENT _____

Appointment Notes

DATE_____   **DOCTOR**_____

Reason for
appointment

_____
_____
_____
_____
_____

Questions to
ask the
doctor

_____
_____
_____
_____
_____

Notes

_____
_____
_____
_____

NEXT APPOINTMENT _____

Appointment Notes

DATE_____   **DOCTOR**_____

Reason for
appointment

_____
_____
_____
_____
_____

Questions to
ask the
doctor

_____
_____
_____
_____
_____
_____

Notes

_____
_____
_____
_____

NEXT APPOINTMENT _____

Appointment Notes

DATE_____   **DOCTOR**_____

Reason for
appointment

_____
_____
_____
_____
_____
_____

Questions to
ask the
doctor

_____
_____
_____
_____
_____
_____
_____

Notes

_____
_____
_____
_____
_____

NEXT APPOINTMENT _____

Appointment Notes

DATE_____   **DOCTOR**_____

Reason for
appointment
_____
_____
_____
_____
_____

Questions to
ask the
doctor
_____
_____
_____
_____
_____
_____

Notes
_____
_____
_____
_____
_____

NEXT APPOINTMENT _____

Appointment Notes

DATE_____ **DOCTOR**_____

Reason for
appointment

_____
_____
_____
_____
_____
_____

Questions to
ask the
doctor

_____
_____
_____
_____
_____
_____

Notes

_____
_____
_____
_____
_____

NEXT APPOINTMENT _____

Appointment Notes

DATE_____   **DOCTOR**_____

Reason for
appointment

_____
_____
_____
_____
_____

Questions to
ask the
doctor

_____
_____
_____
_____
_____
_____

Notes

_____
_____
_____
_____

NEXT APPOINTMENT _____

Appointment Notes

DATE_____ **DOCTOR**_____

Reason for
appointment

_____
_____
_____
_____
_____
_____

Questions to
ask the
doctor

_____
_____
_____
_____
_____
_____

Notes

_____
_____
_____
_____
_____

NEXT APPOINTMENT _____

Appointment Notes

DATE_____   **DOCTOR**_____

Reason for appointment

_____
_____
_____
_____
_____

Questions to ask the doctor

_____
_____
_____
_____
_____
_____

Notes

_____
_____
_____
_____
_____

NEXT APPOINTMENT _____

Appointment Notes

DATE_____ **DOCTOR**_____

Reason for
appointment
_____
_____
_____
_____
_____
_____

Questions to
ask the
doctor
_____
_____
_____
_____
_____
_____
_____

Notes
_____
_____
_____
_____
_____

NEXT APPOINTMENT _____

Appointment Notes

DATE_____   **DOCTOR**_____

Reason for
appointment

_____
_____
_____
_____
_____

Questions to
ask the
doctor

_____
_____
_____
_____
_____
_____

Notes

_____
_____
_____
_____

NEXT APPOINTMENT _____

Appointment Notes

DATE_____   **DOCTOR**_____

Reason for
appointment

_____
_____
_____
_____
_____
_____

Questions to
ask the
doctor

_____
_____
_____
_____
_____
_____

Notes

_____
_____
_____
_____
_____

NEXT APPOINTMENT _____

Appointment Notes

DATE_____   **DOCTOR**_____

Reason for
appointment

_____

_____

_____

_____

_____

_____

Questions to
ask the
doctor

_____

_____

_____

_____

_____

_____

Notes

_____

_____

_____

_____

_____

NEXT APPOINTMENT _____

Appointment Notes

DATE_____ **DOCTOR**_____

Reason for
appointment
_____
_____
_____
_____
_____
_____

Questions to
ask the
doctor
_____
_____
_____
_____
_____
_____

Notes
_____
_____
_____
_____
_____

NEXT APPOINTMENT _____

Appointment Notes

DATE _____   **DOCTOR** _____

Reason for
appointment
_____
_____
_____
_____
_____

Questions to
ask the
doctor
_____
_____
_____
_____
_____
_____

Notes
_____
_____
_____
_____

NEXT APPOINTMENT _____

Appointment Notes

DATE_____   **DOCTOR**_____

Reason for
appointment

_____
_____
_____
_____
_____
_____

Questions to
ask the
doctor

_____
_____
_____
_____
_____
_____

Notes

_____
_____
_____
_____

NEXT APPOINTMENT _____

Appointment Notes

DATE _____   DOCTOR _____

Reason for
appointment

_____
_____
_____
_____
_____

Questions to
ask the
doctor

_____
_____
_____
_____
_____
_____

Notes

_____
_____
_____
_____

NEXT APPOINTMENT _____

Appointment Notes

DATE _____   **DOCTOR** _____

Reason for
appointment
_____
_____
_____
_____
_____
_____

Questions to
ask the
doctor
_____
_____
_____
_____
_____
_____

Notes
_____
_____
_____
_____
_____

NEXT APPOINTMENT _____

Appointment Notes

DATE_____   **DOCTOR**_____

Reason for
appointment

_____
_____
_____
_____
_____

Questions to
ask the
doctor

_____
_____
_____
_____
_____
_____

Notes

_____
_____
_____
_____
_____

NEXT APPOINTMENT _____

Thank You

Made in the USA
Middletown, DE
25 October 2024

63283547R00110